GOUT

EXPLORING ALL THE BASICS OF HEALING GOUT

DR. A. RAMOS

Contents

INTRODUCTION 3

CHAPTER ONE 5

The Identity of the Crystal...5

A Symphony of Indications..7

Restricted range of motion 8

Knowing About Uric Acid 10

The inflammatory reaction 12

CHAPTER TWO 13

Causes and Offenders 14

Trauma or Surgery: 17

Identification..18

Methods of Therapy..23

CHAPTER THREE 28

Nutritional Aspects 28

Drinking plenty of water 30

Modifications to Lifestyle..33

Drinking plenty of water 34

Conclusion...37

THE END 41

INTRODUCTION

A kind of arthritis called gout is typified by the abrupt onset of excruciating pain, swelling, and tenderness in joints, most frequently the big toe. The accumulation of uric acid crystals in the tissues and joints is the cause. Purines are naturally occurring compounds found in some diets and are broken down by the body to produce uric acid.

The body creates too much uric acid or is unable to eliminate it effectively, which causes crystals of excess uric acid to build up in joints and cause excruciating pain and inflammation. If treatment is not received, gout attacks may become more frequent and involve more joints. They can also be intermittent, with intervals of remission.

A diet heavy in purine-rich foods, binge drinking, obesity, certain medical conditions (including renal disease and hypertension), and a family history of gout are risk factors for developing gout. Men are more likely than women to get gout, and the condition tends to become more common as people age.

Dietary adjustments, painkillers, and uric acid-lowering medicines are all part of the management of gout. Persons suffering from gout can lessen the frequency of excruciating attacks by managing their triggers and leading a healthy lifestyle.

CHAPTER ONE

The Identity of the Crystal

Uric acid is the crystal culprit responsible for gout. Purines are compounds that can be found in some meals and are also created by the body. Uric acid is a naturally occurring result of their breakdown. Uric acid dissolves in blood, makes its way to the kidneys, and is eliminated through urine in a healthy person. But this process is interfered with in the case of gout.

Microscopic crystals of excess uric acid occur when the kidneys cannot effectively remove it or when uric acid is produced in excess. These crystals have a tendency to collect in the joints, causing swelling, discomfort, and inflammation all of which are indicative of a gout episode.

These uric acid crystals most frequently form in the big toe joint, but they can also affect the ankles, knees, elbows, wrists, fingers, and other joints. These crystals build up and cause an immunological reaction, which results in the acute, severe gout symptoms.

For the purpose of treating gout, it is essential to comprehend how uric acid crystals contribute to the disease's development. It is frequently advised to alter one's food, lifestyle, and take medicine to lower uric acid levels and stop gout attacks from happening again.

A gout attack's symphony of symptoms produces a crescendo of pain and suffering that is frequently defined by:

Abrupt and Severe Joint Pain:

The main symptom of gout is usually sudden, excruciating joint pain, usually in the big toe. People describe the agony as unbearable, crushing, or throbbing.

Inflammation and Swelling:

The buildup of uric acid crystals and the inflammatory reaction cause the afflicted joint to become swollen, red, and tender.

Redness and Warmth:

There may be a reddish coloring and warmth to the touch in the skin surrounding the injured joint.

A shortened range of motion results from the affected joint's restricted movement brought on by discomfort and edema.

Persistent Unease:

People who have gout may continue to feel dull pain or discomfort in the affected joint even in between acute episodes.

Formation of Tophi:

Gout can cause tophi, or masses of uric acid crystals under the skin, in its severe stages.

Tophi can result in joint abnormalities and are frequently apparent.

Colds and fever:

Fever and chills are possible for certain people, especially in the event of a severe gout attack.

It's crucial to remember that gout symptoms might differ in severity and length. Even though an acute gout attack can be quite painful, it usually goes away in a few days to a week. Gout attacks, however, could return and intensify over time if appropriate care and lifestyle modifications are not taken.

For a precise diagnosis and suitable treatment, it's imperative to contact a doctor if you think you may have gout or exhibit signs of an attack.

The risk of recurring attacks can be decreased and gout can be effectively managed with early intervention and lifestyle changes.

Knowing About Uric Acid

Comprehending the function of uric acid is essential to understanding the mechanics of gout. This is an explanation:

Normal Metabolism of Uric Acid:

Purines, which are substances present in some foods and tissues, naturally break down to produce uric acid as a consequence. The body also produces purines as part of cellular metabolism.

Levels of Uric Acid:

Uric acid dissolves in blood, makes its way to the kidneys, and is eliminated through urine in a healthy person. Sufficient blood levels of uric acid are necessary to keep the body's purine metabolism in equilibrium.

Hyperuricemia in Gout:

Hyperuricemia, or an excess of uric acid in the blood, is the condition that leads to gout. This could be the consequence of either excessive uric acid synthesis or ineffective renal excretion.

Crystallization of Uric Acid:

Microscopic crystals may grow from excess uric acid when levels go too high. These crystals have a tendency to gather in the joints, especially in the body's colder regions, like the big toe joint.

The immune system is triggered by the presence of uric acid crystals in the joints, which results in swelling, discomfort, and inflammation—all of which are indicative of a gout attack.

The following factors can cause hyperuricemia:

Elevated uric acid levels can be caused by a number of things, such as genetics, dietary choices (purine-rich foods, heavy alcohol consumption), certain medical conditions (hypertension, kidney disease), and drugs.

Prolonged Gout:

CHAPTER TWO

Recurrent gout attacks might develop into chronic gout if left untreated. Uric acid crystal buildup over time can result in joint injury and the development of tophi, or masses of uric acid crystals under the skin.

It is crucial to control uric acid levels because of the interaction between uric acid metabolism and the onset of gout. Medication, dietary adjustments, and lifestyle adjustments are frequently used to manage hyperuricemia and stop gout attacks from happening again. Effective gout management and the promotion of general joint health depend heavily on routine monitoring and adherence to treatment regimens.

Finding the triggers for gout attacks is essential to controlling the ailment as there are many potential causes. The following are typical gout culprits and triggers:

Nutritional Decisions:

Foods strong in Purines: Foods strong in purines, like red meat, some vegetables (like asparagus and mushrooms), seafood (like anchovies and sardines), and organ meats (like kidney and liver), can raise uric acid levels.

High-Fructose Corn Syrup: There is a link between consuming high-fructose corn syrup-containing meals or beverages and an elevated risk of gout.

Drinking of Alcohol:

Spirits and Beer: A higher risk of gout has been associated with alcohol consumption, namely beer. Wine and spirits in moderation may also be helpful.

Dehydration:

Dehydration can raise blood uric acid levels, which raises the possibility of crystal formation.

Overweight:

One of the risk factors for gout is being overweight. Elevated levels of uric acid and a higher risk of gout attacks are linked to obesity.

Health Issues:

Hypertension: Gout and high blood pressure frequently coexist.

renal disease: Reduced excretion of uric acid due to impaired renal function can lead to hyperuricemia.

Metabolic Syndrome: Gout may be associated with conditions such as insulin resistance, hypertension, and abdominal obesity.

Drugs:

Uric acid levels can rise with some drugs, such as diuretics (used to treat hypertension).

Genetics:

People may be predisposed to gout if they have a family history of the illness.

Gout attacks can occasionally be triggered by trauma or surgery.

Quick Loss of Weight:

Gout may be brought on by crash diets or abrupt weight loss because they stimulate the body's production of uric acid from bodily tissues.

Age and Gender:

Men are more likely than women to get gout, and the risk rises with age.

Specific Health Events:

Gout episodes can be brought on by infections, acute diseases, or other medical occurrences.

Reducing the frequency of flare-ups and preventing gout attacks need an understanding of and management of these causes. Medication, dietary adjustments, and lifestyle changes can all be used to lower uric acid levels and lessen the effect of gout causes. Gout sufferers should collaborate closely with their medical professionals to create a customized management strategy based on their unique requirements and risk factors.

Identification

A mix of imaging scans, laboratory testing, and clinical evaluations are used to diagnose gout. An outline of the gout diagnosis procedure is provided below:

Clinical Evaluation:

The medical professional will perform a comprehensive physical examination and take a detailed medical history. They will ask about joint pain, swelling, and tenderness, as well as its location, start, and duration. Extreme pain and sudden onset are common features of gout attacks.

Aspiring together (arthrocentesis):

Joint aspiration a procedure in which a tiny needle sample of synovial fluid is taken from the afflicted joint is frequently used to confirm a definitive diagnosis of gout. After that, uric acid crystals are looked for in the fluid using a microscope.

Laboratory Examinations:

Serum Uric Acid Level: Hyperuricemia, or high blood uric acid levels, is linked to gout; however, it's crucial to remember that some gout sufferers may have normal serum uric acid levels in between attacks. Elevated levels by themselves do not provide a diagnosis.

To check for indicators of inflammation, such as an increased white blood cell count, perform a complete blood count (CBC).

Gout attacks may result in elevated levels of C-reactive protein (CRP) and erythrocyte sedimentation rate (ESR), two indicators of inflammation.

Imaging Research:

X-rays: Although they cannot be used to confirm a gout diagnosis, X-rays can be used to rule out other joint conditions or to see the joint damage linked to persistent gout.

Uric acid crystals in the soft tissues and joints can be seen with the use of ultrasound or dual-energy CT scanning.

Clinical Standards:

The presence of particular clinical features, such as the quantity of affected joints, the nature of the attacks, and the presence of tophi, are among the clinical criteria for the classification of gout that have been established by the American College of Rheumatology (ACR).

It is noteworthy that uric acid crystals found during a single episode of joint aspiration are thought to be indicative of gout. However, a combination of clinical criteria, laboratory testing, and imaging studies may be used to establish a diagnosis in situations where joint aspiration is not practical or conclusive.

It is imperative that you seek immediate medical attention if you suspect you have gout or if you are exhibiting symptoms that are consistent with the condition. To find out if gout is the root cause of your joint pain, a medical professional can perform the required examinations and tests.

A combination of dietary adjustments, lifestyle modifications, and medications to regulate uric acid levels, pain, and inflammation are used to treat gout. The following are the main gout treatment modalities:

Drugs:

Nonsteroidal Anti-Inflammatory Drugs (NSAIDs): NSAIDs are frequently prescribed to treat gout attacks by reducing inflammation and relieving pain. Examples of NSAIDs include ibuprofen and naproxen.

Colchicine: The anti-inflammatory drug colchicine is used to treat the symptoms of gout.

When used early on in an attack, it works especially well.

Corticosteroids: To lessen inflammation, corticosteroids may occasionally be prescribed. They can be injected into the injured joint, given orally, or given as an intravenous infusion.

Treatment for Urate-Lowering (ULT):

Allopurinol: Allopurinol is a drug that lowers the body's uric acid production. For the long-term management of gout, it is frequently prescribed to stop recurrent attacks.

Febuxostat: Used as a substitute for allopurinol in cases where a patient is intolerant to the latter, febuxostat inhibits the production of uric acid in a manner similar to that of allopurinol.

Probenecid: Probenecid helps the kidneys excrete more uric acid. It is frequently recommended when urate-lowering drugs are not enough on their own.

Changes in Lifestyle:

Modifications to Diet: Reducing the amount of purine-rich foods, such as shellfish, organ meats, and some vegetables, can help control gout. It's critical to eat a balanced diet and drink plenty of water.

Moderation in Alcohol Use: Reducing alcohol intake, particularly beer and spirits, can lower the risk of gout attacks.

Weight management: Because obesity is a risk factor for gout, it's imperative to reach and maintain a healthy weight through diet and regular exercise.

Handling Acute Attacks:

Rest and elevating the afflicted joint can help during acute gout attacks. Another way to help reduce pain and swelling in the joint is to apply ice to it.

Frequent Observation:

Regular evaluation of total kidney function and uric acid levels is crucial. Medication adjustments might be made in light of patient response to treatment and monitoring results.

Patient Instruction:

Effective long-term management of gout requires educating people about the condition, its triggers, and the significance of medication adherence.

Gout sufferers should collaborate closely with their medical professionals to create a customized treatment plan that addresses their unique requirements and state of health. Successful gout management and a decrease in the frequency of flare-ups are facilitated by routine follow-up appointments and honest communication with medical professionals.

CHAPTER THREE

Nutritional Aspects

Gout management is greatly influenced by diet because it affects uric acid levels. The following food guidelines apply to people who have gout:

Moderation in Foods High in Purines:

Foods high in purines, such as organ meats like liver and kidney, seafood like anchovies, sardines, and mussels, and some vegetables like asparagus and mushrooms, should be consumed in moderation. Moderation is key, but not all foods high in purines need to be avoided.

Trim Proteins:

Lean protein sources like fish, poultry, and tofu are preferable because they produce less uric acid.

Low- or no-fat dairy products:

Select dairy products that are low in fat or fat free, as these have been linked to a decreased risk of gout.

Complex Glycosomics:

Place a focus on complex carbs found in fruits, vegetables, and whole grains. In addition to being nutrient-dense, these foods might also help prevent gout.

Drink plenty of water throughout the day to stay well-hydrated. Sufficient hydration facilitates the excretion of uric acid through urine by diluting it.

Cherries and Products Made from Cherries:

According to some research, cherries and cherry-derived products might have anti-inflammatory qualities and help lower the frequency of gout attacks. Think about including fresh cherries or cherry juice without added sugar in your diet.

Coffee:

Drinking coffee has been linked to a decreased risk of gout. If you drink coffee, consuming it in moderation might be beneficial.

Restricted Consumption of Alcohol:

There is a link between moderate alcohol consumption and a higher risk of gout, particularly with beer and spirits. If you decide to consume alcohol, do so sparingly.

Rich in Vitamin C Foods:

Citrus fruits, strawberries, and bell peppers are among the foods high in vitamin C that may help lower uric acid levels. Think about including these in your diet.

Limit your fructose intake:

Gout risk has been linked to excessive fructose consumption, particularly from high-fructose corn syrup. Pay attention to how much processed food and sugar-filled beverages you consume.

It's crucial to remember that different people react differently to different foods, and that what suits one person may not suit another. Dietary recommendations should also take the person's nutritional requirements and general health into account.

It is best to speak with a medical practitioner or a registered dietitian before making any big dietary changes. To effectively manage gout, they can offer tailored advice based on your unique health status, dietary needs, and preferences.

Certain lifestyle changes, in addition to dietary considerations, can help manage gout and lessen the frequency of flare-ups. Important lifestyle changes for gout sufferers include the following:

Sustain a Healthy Weight:

For those who have gout, achieving and maintaining a healthy weight is essential. Gout is associated with excess body weight, and lowering body weight can help lower uric acid levels.

Frequent Workout:

Regularly partake in mild physical activity to promote general well-being. Engaging in physical activity can aid in managing weight, enhance joint health, and lower the likelihood of gout flare-ups.

Avoid Crash Diets:

Crash diets that cause rapid weight loss may cause bodily tissues to release more uric acid, which could result in gout attacks. Focus on gradual, sustainable weight loss.

Drinking plenty of water

Stay well-hydrated by drinking plenty of water. Hydration helps to dilute uric acid in the blood and promotes its excretion through urine.

Limit Alcohol Intake:

Moderate alcohol consumption, especially of beer and spirits, has been associated with an increased risk of gout. If you decide to consume alcohol, do so sparingly.

Control Your Stress:

Chronic stress can contribute to gout attacks. Explore stress-reducing activities such as meditation, yoga, deep breathing exercises, or hobbies to promote overall well-being.

Quality Sleep:

Ensure you get adequate and quality sleep. Poor sleep patterns and insufficient sleep have been linked to an increased risk of gout attacks.

Foot Care:

Take care of your feet, especially during gout attacks. Avoid putting excessive pressure on the affected joint and consider using supportive footwear.

Regular Medical Check-ups:

Attend regular medical check-ups to monitor uric acid levels and overall health. Discuss any concerns or changes in symptoms with your healthcare provider.

Medication Adherence:

If prescribed medications for gout management, adhere to the recommended dosage and schedule. Report any side effects or changes in symptoms to your healthcare provider.

Educate Yourself:

Learn about gout, its triggers, and effective management strategies. Understanding your condition empowers you to make informed decisions about your lifestyle and treatment plan.

It's important to approach lifestyle adjustments holistically, combining dietary changes, regular exercise, and stress management to effectively manage gout. Consult with your healthcare provider for personalized advice and guidance based on your individual health status and needs.

Conclusion

In conclusion, gout is a form of arthritis characterized by sudden and intense joint pain, swelling, and tenderness, often affecting the big toe. The condition is caused by the buildup of uric acid crystals in the joints, leading to inflammation and debilitating pain.

Managing gout involves a multifaceted approach, combining dietary considerations, lifestyle adjustments, and medications. Dietary changes, such as moderating the intake of purine-rich foods, staying hydrated, and incorporating certain foods like cherries, can help control uric acid levels. Lifestyle adjustments, including maintaining a healthy weight, regular exercise, stress management, and quality sleep, contribute to overall gout management and prevention of flare-ups.

Medications, such as nonsteroidal anti-inflammatory drugs (NSAIDs), colchicine, and urate-lowering therapy (ULT), play a crucial role in relieving symptoms during acute attacks and preventing recurrent episodes. Monitoring uric acid levels, regular medical check-ups, and adherence to treatment plans are essential components of long-term gout management.

Education and awareness about gout, its triggers, and effective management strategies empower individuals to take an active role in their health. By adopting a comprehensive and personalized approach, individuals with gout can lead fulfilling lives with reduced pain and improved joint health.

If you suspect you have gout or are experiencing symptoms, it's important to seek timely medical attention for an accurate diagnosis and tailored treatment plan. Working closely with healthcare professionals ensures effective gout management and an improved quality of life.

THE END

www.ingramcontent.com/pod-product-compliance
Lightning Source LLC
Chambersburg PA
CBHW070745260726
48660CB00007B/2992